THE PRITIKIN DIET FOR BEGINNERS."

"Transform Your Health with The Pritikin Diet: Healthy living – a beginner's blueprint for heart healthy living and sustainable wellbeing.

OPTIMALWELLNESS

TABLE OF CONTENT

INTRODCION

WHAT IS THE PRITIKIN DIET

ADVANTAGES OF PRITIKIN DIET

GETTING STARTED ESSENCIAL TIPS FOR THE BEGINNER

BENEFITS OF THE PRITIKIN DIET:

CHAPTER ONE

 PRITIKIN DIET BASICS

UNDERSTANDING THE PRITIKIN PRINCIPLE

THE SCIENCE BEHIND THE PRITIKIN DIET

FOOD TO INCLUDE AND AVOID

CHAPTER 2

 SETTING UP UR KITTCHEN

1 STOCKING YOUR PANTRY WITH PRITIKIN FRIENDLY STAMPLES

ESSENTIAL KITCHEN TOOLS AND EQUIPMENT

<u>CHAPTER3</u>

 BREAKFAST RECIPES

ENERGIZING MORNING SMOOTHIES

OATMEAL VARIATIONS

WHOLE GRAIN PANCAKES

SCRAMBLES AND OMELETS

<u>CHAPTER 4</u>

 LUNCH IDEALSFRESH AND FILLING SALADS

PLANT-BASED SANDWICHES AND BURGERS

<u>CHAPTER 5</u>

 DINNER DELIGHTS

LEAN PROTEIN ENTRESS

HOME MADE SAUCES AND DRESSINGS

<u>CHAPTER 6</u>

SNACKS AND APPETIZERS

NUTRIENT PACKED SNACK IDEAS

PARTY- READY APPETIZER

CHAPTER 7

DESSERTS AND TREATS

SWEET ENDING WITH A HEALTHY TWIST

FRUIT BASED DESSERTS

GUILT—FREE BAKING

CHAPTER 8

MEAL PLANNING AND PREPPING

WEEKLY MEAL PLANS

TRACKING PROGRESS AND HEALTH BENEFITS

CONCLUSION

INTRODCTION

INTRODCTION

Nathan Pritikin developed it the late 1970s, and it is a diet-and-lifestyle program called the Pritikin Diet. This diet is centered around whole foods and a low-fat, low-cholesterol diet. Pritikin Diet strives to enhance cardiac fitness, reduce body fat mass (BIM), and improve general health and vigor.

HERE'S A BRIEF INTRODUCTION TO THE KEY PRINCIPLES OF THE PRITIKIN DIET FOR BEGINNERS:

1. **Whole Foods Emphasis**: One such diet is the Pritikin which focuses on eating whole, unrefined foods comprising fruits, vegetables, whole grains, beans, and lean meat. They contain all vital nutrients and fiber.

2. **Low-Fat, Low-Cholesterol**: These include taking the least amount of saturated fats, trans fats and dietary cholesterol. It refers to meat selection, cutting down on foods prepared with too much oil, and using cooking processes such as broiling, steaming amongst others.

3. Limiting Processed Foods: Sugar, salt and saturated fat are commonly added in processed foods so these products are not recommended on the Pritikin diet. On the contrary, people are advised to concentrate on their natural and pure alternative.

4. Portion Control: Nevertheless, portions are another important part of the Pritikin diet which places the main focus on all wholesome and nutritious foods. Controlling ones' weight by managing portion sizes and preventing.

size helps in controlling weight and prevents overeating.

5. Regular Exercise: Physical exercise, alongside the Pritikin diet. This exercise forms an important aspect in overall health and control of bodyweight.

6. Hydration: The Pritikin lifestyle encourages adequate water intake. Drinking a lot of water helps one achieve good health and also makes one feel full such that it might be instrumental in managing weight.

7. Scientific Foundation: The Pritkin Diet has its origins in science, especially when it comes to heart disease. The program is aimed at reducing chances of getting coronary attacks as well as alteration of other health indicators using diet based remedies.

A medical doctor or a registered dietician should be consulted before embarking on any new diet or lifestyle programs. This helps them offer customized counseling depending on their health requirements and aspirations. Moreover, one could note that people's tastes and health state can be taken into account in adjusting the Pritikin Diet to a particular person.

Pritikin's Diet is rich in fruits, vegetables, whole grains, and lean meats and has lower amounts of fat. It was called the Pronto diet or simply "Prato". While individual responses to diets can vary,

Here are some potential advantages associated with the Pritikin Diet:

1. Heart Health: The pritikin diet has been specially created to ensure heart safety by concentrating only on very low-fat as well as very low-cholesterol foods. This might assist in reducing blood pressure, cholesterol levels and improving general cardiac wellbeing.

2. Weight Loss: Many people will lose their weight by eating fewer calories in comparison with processed food. It fosters low calorie and high fiber foods which leave one satisfied.

3. Improved Blood Sugar Control: Eating whole grains, fruits, and vegetables such as those found in a Pritikin Diet may help balance blood sugar levels. It is especially important for diabetics or people susceptible to diabetes.

4. Rich in Nutrients: Such a diet should comprise of whole, minimally processed foods with vitamins, minerals, and antioxidants important for the body. It may assist in promoting general health and wellness.

5. Sustainable: The Pritikin Diet is not a short-term, restricted eating plan but it encompasses a lifelong healthy living lifestyle. However, this would be more sustainable for some people since it does not require severe limitations or denial practices.

6. Support for Overall Health: This diet is meant to enhance general health and improve weight. Also, it enables nutrition balance and also encourages healthy food intake linked to multiple health benefits.

7. Lifestyle Education: In some cases, the Pritikin Program is accompanied by an educative part about exercise, stress and so on with a view to having these lifestyle factors change along with the change in the diet to promote a wholesome well-being.

However, it is very important to bear in mind that different people respond differently to various diet programmers; hence, a diet which will work fine for someone might not be beneficial to another. The fact is that you must see a doctor before changing your diet significantly, especially if you are sick. Moreover, nutrition is an evolving domain with emerging data that can possibly indicate long-term limitations and advantages of selected foods.

Support for Overall Health: Overall health and wellness are factored in while the diet focuses on more than just losing weight. The diet promotes balanced nutrition and consuming food that is beneficial for different aspects of your health.

If you're considering starting the Pritikin Diet, here are some essential tips for beginners:

1. **Educate Yourself:** It is important to consider where an individual is coming from. Find out what the Pritikin diet is made up about and how eating should be like when adhered to this plan.

2.**Focus on Whole Foods:** In the case of Pritikin Diet, it entails consumption of whole unmodified foods. Choose more items such as vegetables, fruits, whole grains, lean proteins. Eating less of processed or refined food.

3. **Low-Fat,** High-Fiber Choices: Choose foods with less saturate and trans fat. Take in adequate fiber rich foods such as whole grains, legumes, fruits, and vegetables among others. Satisfies hunger, it is also good for digestion in fibers.

4. **Lean Proteins**: Select leaner proteins like chicken, sea food, and beans/legumes. Include low fat red meat and processed meats because they are high in saturated fats.

5. **Portion Control:** This entails eating foods that are in their whole, but one should also make sure he or she observes portion control. Make sure that you do not eat too much just because a food is healthy.

6. **Limit Added Sugars and Salt**: Limit intake of sugary and salty food and drinks. These include soft drinks, junk food among many others that are full of sugar.

7. **Stay Hydrated**: Make sure you drink enough water during the entire day. Drinking water is important for general good health, and it may also be used as a means of feeling satiated.

8. **Gradual Transition**: Instead of making drastic changes all at once, you should go ahead and do it step by step. This enhances the sustainability of adjustments.

9. **Meal Planning**: Plan your meals ahead of time to ensure that you have a variety of Pritikin-friendly foods available. This can help you avoid relying on less healthy options when you're hungry and in a rush.

10. **Physical Activity:** The Pritikin Program often includes an emphasis on regular physical activity. Find activities you enjoy and aim for a balance of cardiovascular exercise, strength training, and flexibility exercises.

11. **Consult a Professional**: Before making significant changes to your diet, especially if you have existing health conditions, consult with a healthcare professional or a registered dietitian. They can provide personalized advice based on your individual needs and health status.

12. **Track Your Progress**: Keep track of your meals, physical activity, and any changes you observe in your health. This can help you stay motivated and make adjustments as needed.

1. Heart Health

- Researchers have found that those on the Pritikin Diet tend to have lower cholesterols and a decreased risk of heart problems as well.

2. Weight Management

- It also contributes towards promoting a healthy weight, through its focus on whole foods and low caloric density foods.

3. Blood Pressure Control

- This diet emphasizes on having low sodium foods that may lead to effective management of blood pressure.

4. Diabetes Prevention

- Eating whole foods that are also low fat may help prevent and manage type 2 diabetes.

5. Overall Well-being

• A healthy lifestyle in which you consume nutritious food and engage in exercise promotes sound general health. It also boosts your stamina and makes you happier.

• Chooses complex carbohydrates instead of simple sugars.

CHAPTER ONE

PRITIKIN DIET BASICS

Pritikin diet is a low fat, high fiber diet formulated by Nathan Prikin in the 1970's. It serves for improving the heart condition, losing excess weight and general health.

Here are the basic principles of the Pritikin Diet

<u>Emphasis on Whole, Plant-Based Foods</u>:

1. The cornerstone of Pritikin diet is made up of whole and raw foods from plants. These consist of fruits, vegetables, brown rice, beans, nuts, and seeds.
2. All these foods contain important elements like vitamins, dietary fibers, essential minerals, and antioxidants.

<u>Low in Saturated and Trans Fats:</u>

1. Saturated and trans fats are minimized in Pritikin diet, they are mostly associated with

animal products and processed foods. They minimize high-fat dairy, fatty meats, and fried foods.

They include healthy fats from moderate's sources of avocado, nuts and olive oil.

Lean Protein Sources:

1. Lean protein sources include poultry, fish, legumes, tofu, and tempeh.

2. High-fat red meat and processed meats are limited because of their high content in saturated fats.

High-Fiber Foods:

1. Eating foods with high levels of dietary fiber is encouraged especially foods like whole grains, fruits, vegetables, as well as legumes.
2. Fiber promotes satiety so you don't get hunger pangs after your meal, helps in digestion, and generally provides the cardiovascular benefits of fiber.

Limitation of Added Sugars and Salt:

1. Specifically, it forbids the intake of those drinks and foods containing high added sugars like sweeteners. These include soft drinks, chocolates, and candy bars.
2. Heart health is supported by also discouraging excessive salt intake. There is also limited amount of processed food that contains high levels of added salts.

Portion Control:

1. Although it focuses more on nutrient dense food, a Pritikin diet considers that one should eat in appropriate portions. This assists in controlling how many calories are taken in one sitting.

Hydration:

1. Nathan Pritikin has created in the 1970's a low fat, high fiber diet called the Pritikin diet. Heart health, weight loss, and a

general feeling of wellness are promoted by it.

Emphasis on Whole, Plant-Based Foods:

1. The bases of the Pritkin diet are made up of natural whole grain and plant based foods. They are fruits, vegetables, whole grains, legumes, nuts, and seeds.
2. It constitutes of vital nutrients like vitamin, minerals, antioxidant and fibre.

Low in Saturated and Trans Fats:

1. The Pritikin Diet consists of minimal fat amounts including saturated and trans fats that are mostly found in animal products as well as refined goods. These reduce consumption of high-fat dairy, fatty meats, and fried foods.
2. However, healthy fat such as from nut, avocado and olive oil is taken in moderate amount.

Lean Protein Sources:

1. Lean protein sources include poultry, fish, legumes, tofu, and tempeh.

2. They are high in saturated fats, hence, the limit of red meats and processed meats.

High-Fiber Foods:

- These foods include whole grains, fresh fruits, vegetables, and beans.
- It also promotes satiety, facilitates digestion, and supports general cardiovascular health.

Hydration:

1. Overall, healthy life is encouraged through adequate water intake. Digestion is stimulated by water, metabolism is also helped by it and it is healthier compared to sugar-laden fluids.

Regular Physical Activity:

1. Normally, a Pritikin Program can incorporate routine exercise. In fact, regular physical activity or exercise could

be looked upon as a critical ingredient in ensuring total fitness and good health.

Gradual Transition:

1. Many people advise that people should change their diets slowly instead of going suddenly from not eating much at all to being on a diet. Such a move will make the process more lasting for years.

Lifestyle Education:

1. Education is usually not limited to just one factor but lifestyle related issues such as stress management and sleep are included in the program making it a holistic diet plan.

2. However, some people could take that particular diet with a doctor's recommendation in case they already had existing health problems. One should

seek medical advice prior any major shift in diet.

3. the Pritikin Diet is just an option of a general healthy diet response differs from one person to another. However, before making major changes to your diet, you should probably go see a doctor or a registered dietician to check if this is the right diet for you.

The Pritikin Principle is a nomenclature for the code and way of life that belongs to the Pritikin Program initiated by Nathan Pritikin. In general, the purpose of the Pritikin Principle should be aimed at improving cardiovascular health and promoting weight management.

Here are key aspects of the Pritikin Principle:

1.   **Whole, Plant-Based Foods:**
   - The Pritikin Principle promotes more intake of whole and natural vegetables and fruits. These consist of fruits, vegetables, whole grains, beans, nuts and seeds.
   - They contain such necessary substances as vitamins, fiber, and antioxidants which make up people's organism.

2.   **Low in Saturated and Trans Fats:**

- This principle advocates for taking foods with low levels of saturated and trans fats. It means consuming less fatty foods from animals with minimal processing or frying of foods.

3.   **Lean Proteins:**

- The principle emphasizes on consuming lean proteins like fishes, poultry and legumes, as well as products derived from plant proteins. Limit of red meat and processed meats include high saturated fat content.

4.   **High-Fiber Foods:**

- The dietary fiber, which constitutes a very significant aspect of Pritikin Principle, has been highlighted above. A high fiber diet comprises of whole grain foods, fruits, vegetables, beans among many more other foods which facilitate proper digestion, stabilize blood sugar, and promote feelings of satiation.

5. **Limitation of Added Sugars and Salt:**
   - The idea is that one should avoid consuming diets and drinks that are sugar-rich. Such foods containing excess salts are restricted to avoid heart diseases.

6. **Portion Control:**
   - The diet also focuses on portion control and encourages nutrient-dense foods so that you don't consume too many calories. It also assists people in achieving healthy weights.

7. **Hydration:**
   - The principle urges adequate water intake. Water is of benefit to one's health and good for your digestive system than consuming sweet beverages

Regular Physical Activity:

- In this sense, the Pritikin Principle includes daily exercise as part of a healthy way of life. It is known that exercise is very important for cardiovascular health, diet control, and general good health.

8.   **Lifestyle Education:**

- Education on different lifestyle issues is common in the Pritikin program. This would include stress handling, quality sleep, among many healthy habits for general wellbeing.

9. **Gradual Transition:**

- People are discouraged from fast diet or exercise change as they have to slowly change the entire diet and lifestyle. It is assumed that this gradual approach will sustain the transition on a longer time basis.

10.   **Medical Supervision:**

- These include low-fat diets that are rich in protein and high in fiber. This entails cutting down on the consummation of animal fatty products while limiting the intake of processed and fast food items.

11.   Lean Proteins:

- However, the diet is based on the Pritikin Principle which emphasizes on lean protein such as poultry, fish, beans or even other vegetarian sources of protein. This arises because red meat and processed meats have a low unsaturated-to-saturated fat ratio, making them unhealthy for consumption in large quantities.

12.   High-Fiber Foods:

- Pritikin Principle involves dietary fiber. Diet also consists of high-fiber foods like whole grains, fruits, vegetables, and legumes for good digestion, blood sugar control, and satisfaction.

13.   Limitation of Added Sugars and Salt:

- This principle encourages avoiding such high-sugar foods and drinks. Limitation of highly-salt processed foods is recommended for cardiac benefits.

14.   Portion Control:

- On the other hand, the Pritikin Principle requires proper portion controls for the limited consumption of energy provided by these foods. This aids people in maintaining an ideal body weight.

15.   Hydration:

- One of the principles encourages individuals to take enough water into their bodies. Overall, water promotes health, aids in digestion, and is a better option than carbonated beverages.

Pritikin Diet is built up on scientifically based facts about the cardio vascular system, the weight control and health problems in general. There are researches done into individual diets and how they affect health for example.

Here are some key scientific aspects behind the Pritikin Diet:

1. **Low-Fat, High-Fiber Approach:**
   - Research indicates that diets rich in fibers could lower blood cholesterol and decrease the risk of heart disease. A diet with such an emphasis could lower cholesterol, lower blood pressure, and support heart health in general.

2. **Plant-Based Nutrition:**
   - Many researches reveal that plant based diets promote healthy living. Plant based diets decrease risk of cardiovascular diseases, type 2 diabetes and some cancers. These health-related benefits result from the high levels of antioxidants

and phytochemicals found in plant-based foods.

3. **Whole Grains and Blood Sugar Control**:
   - A hallmark of all dietary programs is consumption of high-grade whole grains, which is well known to possess a much smaller glycemic index than do refined grains. It may help in blood sugar control thereby making the diet advantageous for people living with diabetes and those with higher risks of becoming diabetic.

4. **Lean Proteins and Weight Management:**
   - This is based on studies showing such diets help maintain muscle and manage calories. Saturation is also associated with protein.

5. **Hydration and Health:**
   - Research indicates that ample drinking water should be taken to support the Pritikin Diet since it helps in promoting

physical wellness. Water plays an important role in many physiological processes such as digestion, transport of nutrients as well as regulation of body temperature.

6. **Exercise and Cardiovascular Health:**
   - Physical exercise is one of the central elements of the Pritikin Program. It is also proven by scientific evidence that exercise is good for health of heart, weight management as well as general wellness.

7. **Behavioral Changes and Sustainability:**
   - The Pritikin Principle emphasizes that healthy change should happen slowly and last long. # Behavioral research psychologists agree that long-term small-step changes are better than overnight big shots.

8. **Clinical Studies and Outcomes:**

- The Pritikin Longevity Center, established by Nathan Pritikin, has undertaken and published research on Pritikin Program efficacy. The studies have shown beneficial effects including those on cardiovascular health, weight loss, and several others.

However, one should keep in mind that although science supports the fundamentals of the Pritikin Diet, individual responses to diet may differ. The discipline of nutritional science also changes all the time, with new discoveries being made every day regarding food and well-being. However, when it comes to serious dieting, especially if you have a medical condition like this, you ought to see a doctor or a dietician first so as to receive tailored recommendation that is right for you.

The Pritikins Diet centers whole non adulterated foodstuffs that are designed to enhance cardiac system life and general wellbeing.

Here are general guidelines for foods to include and avoid in the Pritikin Diet:

Foods to Include:

1. **Fruits:**
   - Consider some fresh and raw fruits. Examples of these are berries, citrus fruit, apple and banana.

2. **Vegetables:**
   - Eat as many different colored vegetables as possible. It is important to include a variety such as dark leafy greens, cabbage, hot peppers, or tomatoes among others.

3. **Whole Grains:**
   - Select healthy whole grain products like brown rice, quinoa, barley, oatmeal, or whole wheat. This is obtained from these that are source of fiber and nutrients.

4. **Legumes:**
   - The addition of legumes can consist of beans, peens, and lentils. They make good plant-based protein and fiber.

5. **Aleena Proteins:**
   - Choose lean proteins such as skinless poultry, fish, tofu, tempeh or beans. Control intake of red meat and avoid processed meats.

6. **Nuts and Seeds:**
   - Provide moderate percentages of nuts and seeds including almonds, walnuts, chia seeds, and flaxseeds. They are healthy fats that contain the needed minerals.

7. **Dairy or Dairy Alternatives:**
- Select dairy products that are low in fat or no fat such as yogurt, skimmed milk. However, you can use almond milk and soy milk which is a good alternative from dairy products.

8. **Healthy Fats:**
- Use healthy fats sparingly, for example those from an avocado or olive oil.

9. **Herbs and Spices:**
- Instead of using excess salt or sugar, use herbs and other spices to make your food tasty.

10. **Water:**
- Therefore, keep yourself adequately hydrated by taking a lot of pure water.

1. **Processed and Refined Foods**:
   - Reduce the intake of processed and refined products, such as sugar confectionaries, soda drinks and sweetened corn.

2. **Added Sugars:**

Reduce consumption of drinks and foods containing added sugar. Sodas, sweetened juices, and desserts are some of them.

3. **High-Fat Dairy:**
   - Restrict high fat dairy food like whole milk and whole cheese. Ensure you go for lower-fat and fat-free options.

4. **Red and Processed Meats:**
   - Cut down on consumption of red meat such as bacon, sausages, etc., and, avoid eating foods with additives.

5. **Fried Foods:**
   - Some fried foods contain excessive amounts of bad cholesterol that cause heart problems; therefore, these particular foods should be avoided or at least eaten very little.

6. **Excess Salt:**
   - Using less salt as an additive. Beware of processed foods which might contain excessive amount of salt.

7. **Highly Processed Snacks:**
   - Keep highly processed snacks such as crisps, biscuits, and cookies at bay.

9. **Butter and Lard:**
   - Use butter and lard sparingly. Use healthier cooking oils such as olive oil instead.

CHAPTER 2

SETTING UP UR KITTCHEN

To cater for Pritikin diet, one needs to fill his/her kitchen with whole fresh foods.

Here are some tips to help beginners set up their kitchens for the Pritikin Diet:

1. **Stock Up on Fresh Produce**:

 Fruits: Apples, bananas, berries, citrus fruits.

Vegetables: Spinach, leafy greens, broccoli, cauliflower, carrots, and peppers.

2. **Whole Grains:**

Brown Rice, Quinoa, Barley, Oats: They form bases of many meals.

3. **Legumes**:

Beans, Lentils, Chickpeas: Dry beans and peas are great sources of vegetable protein and fiber.

4.   **Lean Proteins:**

Skinless Poultry, Fish, Tofu, Tempeh: Include lean proteins like fish and chicken in your meals.

5.   **Nuts and Seeds:**

Almonds, Walnuts, Chia Seeds, Flaxseeds: They are healthy fats that can be sprinkled over salads or yogurt.

6.   **Dairy or Dairy Alternatives:**

Low-Fat or Fat-Free Dairy, Plant-Based Milk: Go for food items that have lower saturated fats levels.

7.   **Healthy Fats:**

Avocados, Olive Oil: They can be used in cooking or as salads.

8.   **Herbs and Spices:**

Garlic, Basil, Cilantro, Turmeric: Buy a lot of herbs and spices which you can use to give some flavor to your meals without adding too much salt.

9.   Whole Wheat Products:

Whole Wheat Bread, Pasta, and Brown Rice: They are sources of complex carbohydrates and fiber.

10.   Minimize Processed Foods:

Limit or Avoid: It includes processed snacks, candy bars, sugar rich cereals and heavily processed frozen meals.

11.   Food Storage Containers:

Purchase large and microwave safe containers for making meals in advance and storing leftover food.

12.   Kitchen Tools:

Steamer: Can be applied while cooking vegetables that do not cause loss of nutrients.

Blender: Good mixing bowl for making fruit and vegetable smoothies.

Food Scale: Helps with portion control.

13.   Water Filtration System:

Get clean, filtered water for you.

14.   Educational Resources:

Consider using inspirational and guiding sources such as cookbooks, online resources, and meal plans that follow the Pritikin Diet.

15.   Meal Planning Tools:

Organize your weekly meals and write out grocery list on a white board or planner.

16.   Label Reading:

The key is learning to read food labels and identifying added sugars, unhealthy fats, and high salt content.

17.   Non-Stick Cookware:

Try using non-stick pans or cooking methods such as steaming or baking instead of frying.

18.   Mindful Eating Environment:

To encourage mindful eating, create a comfortable and pleasant dining area.

19.   Health Monitoring Tools:

You can try using a weighing balance, measuring cups, among others for proper portion control.

20.   Regular Grocery Shopping:

Visit a local grocery store at least once every couple of weeks to get fresh vegetables and some of the necessary supplies.

Understand that assimilating a different diet may take some time, and hence, it is good to bear with yourself during the process. The kitchen should be well-planned and stocked accordingly for easy work in case one wants to do it continuously and find the job more enjoyable. Get an appointment with a Registered Dietician or nutrition professionals for bespoke advice if you can.

One of the first things you need to do when going the Pritikin way involves stocking your pantry with basic Pritikin diet friendly staples.

Here's a list of pantry essentials that align with the principles of the Pritikin Diet:

Grains and Cereals:

1. Brown Rice
2. Quinoa
3. Barley
4. Steel-Cut Oats
5. Whole Wheat Pasta
6. Low-added sugar Whole Grain Cereals

Legumes and Pulses:

1. Beans – canned or dried (black, kidney, cannellini, etc.).
2. Lentils
3. Chickpeas
4. Split Peas

<u>**Nuts and Seeds:**</u>

1. Almonds
2. Walnuts
3. Flaxseeds
4. Sunflower Seeds

<u>**Oils and Fats:**</u>

1. Extra Virgin Olive Oil
2. Canola Oil
3. Avocado Oil

<u>**Herbs, Spices, and Seasonings**</u>:

1. Garlic
2. Onion
3. Basil
4. Cilantro
5. Turmeric
6. Cumin
7. Coriander
8. Paprika
9. Black Pepper

<u>**Canned Goods**</u>:

1. Tomato Sauce (low sodium)
10.   Diced Tomatoes (no added salt)
11.   Low-Sodium Vegetable Broth
12.   Tuna, canned, packed in water; or, Salmon.

<u>**Condiments and Sauces:**</u>

1. Mustard (without added sugars)
2. Apple Cider Vinegar
3. Soy Sauce (low sodium)
4. Salsa (without added sugars)

<u>**Whole Grains and Baking:**</u>

1. Whole Wheat Flour
2. Whole Wheat Tortillas
3. Baking Powder
4. Baking Soda

Snacks:

1. Air-Popped Popcorn
2. Rice Cakes
3. Unsalted Rice Crackers

Sweeteners:

1. Stevia
2. Agave Nectar

Beverages:

1. Herbal Teas
3. Coffee
4. Water

Miscellaneous:

1. Low-Sodium Ketchup
2. Dijon Mustard
3. Low-Fat Salad Dressings

Kitchen Essentials:

1. Food Storage Containers
2. Measuring Cups and Spoons
3. Non-Stick Cooking Spray

4. Types of spoons and utensils available.
5. A Good Set of Knives

Educational Resources:
1. Pritikin Diet Cookbook or Recipes
2. Nutrition Books or Guides

Meal Planning Tools:
1. Weekly Meal Planning can be done using the Whiteboard or Planner.

Health Monitoring Tools:

1. Food Scale
2. Measuring Cups

Specialty Items (Optional):

1. E.g., Brown Rice Pasta.
2. Quinoa Flour
3. Nutritional Yeast

Ensure you read labels for extra salt, sugars, and nasty fats when opting for packs. Also, ensure that you go for diversity of options you make so as to attain balanced diet. It is important to keep on stocking up the pantry staples in order to ensure there is always adequate, crisp and healthy ingredients at hand. Consult the services of a registered dietician, should there be an opportunity. The latter will advise you accordingly on meals appropriate for you.

ESSENTIAL KITCHEN TOOLS AND EQUIPMENT

One of the useful strategies in preparing meals for you is to set up your kitchen with appropriate tools.

Here's a list of essential kitchen tools for beginners following the Pritikin Diet:

1.   **Cutting Board:**

Opt for hard cutting board used to cut fruit, vegetables, and lean proteins.

2.   **Chef's Knife:**

Buy a good quality chef's knife for ease of cutting.

3.   **Paring Knife:**

A smaller knife for fine cuttings such as trimming and peeling.

4.   **Vegetable Peeler:**

Can be used for peeling of fruits like sweet potato, cucumber etc.

5. **Blender:**

Best for blending of fruits and vegetables in smoothies.

6. **Food Processor:**

Well-suited for chopping, slicing, preparing salads and serving sauce/dip.

7. **Steamer Basket:**

To cook vegetables with no loss of nutrients.

8. **Non-Stick Skillet or Pan:**

Go for the non-stick and lightly oiled cook.

9. **Saucepan:**

Necessary for cooking of grains, legumes or sauces.

10. **Baking Sheets:**

They are used on vegetable roasting's and baking whole grain.

11.   Measuring Cups and Spoons:

It is vital that measures be as accurate as possible, if a recipe is to be followed.

12. Mixing Bowls:

Sizes of mixing ingredients, tossing salads, etc.

3. Colander:

Drain cooked pasta and vegetables.

14. Salad Spinner:

Efficiently washes and dries salad greens.

15. Tongs

Perfect at all times especially when trying to flip foods during cooking.

16. Can Opener:

To open a can of a product like beans or tomatoes.

17. Pepper Grinder:

The dish is seasoned with freshly ground black pepper.

18. Herb and Spice Rack:

Arrange your most used herbs and spices in this order for easy accessibility.

19. Citrus Juicer:

Squeeze out fresh juice from lemons, limes, and oranges.

20. Digital Food Scale:

Assist in portion control and specific ingredient portions.

21. Mixing Utensils:

Spatulas, whisk and wooden as well as silicon spoon.

22. Non-Stick Cooking Spray:

Cut down on uncalled for cooking oil usage.

23. Water Filtration Pitcher:

Provide ready access to clean filtrated water.

24. Storage Containers:

Preserve leftovers and pre-meal ingredients.

25. Whiteboard or Planner:

Plan your menu for the week and shopping list.

26. Nut Milk Bag or Cheesecloth:

Homemade nut milk or juice straining."

27. Instant-Read Thermometer:

I keep my meats at ideal cooking temperatures.

28. Salad Dressing Shaker:

Manufacture your own dressings.

29. Microplate Grater:

Serrated for grating of garlic, ginger, or citrus.

30. Kitchen Timer:

Helps with precise cooking times.

Always ensure that you keep replacing and maintaining your kitchen tools as often is necessary. As you follow the Pritikin, having the correct equipment can allow you to enjoy your cooking experience better, making it quicker.

CHAPTER 3

BREAKFAST RECIPES

Below, I will give some breakfast recipes that will work good for those who are just starting their diet on the Pritikin way. These recipes focus on whole, unprocessed foods, and are designed to provide a nutritious start to your day:

1. Oatmeal with Berries and Nuts:

Ingredients:

- 1/2 cup steel-cut oats
- 1 cup water
- half a cup of mixed berry mix consisting of strawberry, blueberry and raspberry.
- Chopped one tablespoon of almonds or nuts.
- 1 teaspoon ground flaxseeds

Instructions:

- Follow cooking instructions indicated on package for oatmeal in a cup of water.

- Sprinkle on your choice of mixed berries, chopped nuts, or ground flaxseeds on top.

2. Fruit and Yogurt Parfait:

Ingredients:

- 1 cup of low-fat or fat-free Greek yogurt
- 1/3 cup chopped mango/pineapple apple/
- low-sugar granola, ¼ cup
- 1 tablespoon chia seeds

Instructions:

- Put layers of Greek yogurt, diced fruits, and some granola in a glass or a bowl.
- Add texture by sprinkling some more Chia seeds.

3. Whole Grain Toast with Avocado and Tomato:

INGREDIENTS:

- 2 slices whole grain bread
- 1/2 avocado, mashed

- 1 small tomato, sliced
- Salt and pepper to taste
- Optional: a pinch or two of red pepper flakes

Instructions:

- Heat the toast over wholegrain bread.
- Layer your mashed avocado across the toast nicely.
- Top with sliced tomatoes. Add a little bit of salt, peppered, and hot red pepper flakes.

4. Vegetable Omelets:

Ingredients:

- 2 eggs (or egg whites)
- 1/4 cup diced bell peppers
- 1/4 cup diced tomatoes
- 1/4 cup chopped spinach
- Salt and pepper to taste
- Optional: a spoon of feta cheese – moderate quantity.

Instructions:

- Combine eggs in a bowl, salt, pepper, then whisk.
- Sauté the bell peppers, tomatoes, and spinach in a non-stick pan until tender.
- Add the whisked eggs on top of the vegetables and cook until the omelets is done.
- Optional: Sprinkle with feta cheese.

5. Smoothie Bowl:

Ingredients:

- 1 cup frozen mixed berries
- 1/2 banana
- Half a cup of non-fat or reduced-fat Greek yogurt.
- 1 tablespoon chia seeds
- Toppings: sliced strawberries, granola, honey drizzle (optional)

INSTRUCTIONS:

- Mix the frozen berries, banana and Greek yoghurt until they are smooth.
- Place them in a bowl and finish with a sprinkle of chai seeds, sliced strawberries, and granola.
- Optional: Drizzle with honey for sweetness.

6. Chia Seed Pudding:

Ingredients:

- tablespoons chia seeds
- Half a cup of preferred milk, e.g., almond milk.
- 1/2 teaspoon vanilla extract
- Toppings: banana slices, berries, with a pinch of cinnamon

INSTRUCTIONS:

- Put chia seeds, almond milk, and vanilla in a bowl.
- Place in a refrigerator and let rest for more than two hours until thickened.
- Serve with bananas, berries topped with cinnamon.

You should consider these as just a few examples of how one could create breakfast recipes based on what is appealing to one's taste buds. In case of any special health concerns, it is advisable to seek advice from a doctor or dietician before embarking on major food adjustments.

Certainly! Here are a few energizing morning smoothie recipes that align with the principles of the Pritikin Diet:

1. Berry Bliss Smoothie:

Ingredients:

- one cup of mixed berries including strawberries, blueberries, and raspberries
- 1/2 banana
- Half a cup of low-fat or fat-free Greek yogurt
- 1 tablespoon chia seeds
- Half a cup of water or almond milk
- Ice cubes (optional)

Instructions:

- Blend all ingredients until smooth.
- If you want something cold, add some ice cubes.

2. Green Power Smoothie:

Ingredients:

- 1 cup spinach
- 1/2 cucumber, peeled and sliced
- Halved and chopped green apple without seeds.
- 1/2 lemon, juiced
- Half a cup of water or coconut water
- Ice cubes (optional)

Instructions:

- Mix together spinach, cucumber, green apple, and lemonade in a blender until it is completely pureed.
- Lastly, add water or coco water then re-blend.
- Add ice cubes if desired.

1. Tropical Paradise Smoothie:

Ingredients:

- 1/2 cup pineapple chunks

- 1/2 mango, peeled and diced
- 1/2 banana
- one-half cup of low-fat or nonfat Greek yogurt
- 1 tablespoon flaxseeds
- Alternatively, a person can use half a cup of either coconut nut or almond.
- Ice cubes (optional)

Instructions:

- Mix banana, cocoa powder, Greek yoghurt, and almond butter into a consistent mixture.
- Puree in some water or almond milk if you wish.
- Add ice cubes if desired.

These simple smoothie recipes offer lots of minerals and vitamins that you might want to suit with yours tasting needs. Try various fruits, greens, and liquid bases to discover the best of them for yourself. Always make sure you serve the right amounts of food for your diet

Certainly! Oatmeal is one of the most flexible as well as nourishing breakfast item for those who are following the Pritikin diet program.

Here are some oatmeal variations for beginners following the Pritikin Diet:

1. Mixed Berry Oatmeal:

Ingredients:

- 1/2 cup steel-cut oats
- 1 cup water
- Half a cup of mixed berries including strawberries, blackberries, and blueberries
- A teaspoon of cut nuts (almonds or walnut).
- 1 teaspoon chia seeds

Instructions:

- Cook as per pack instructions of steel cut oats in water.

- Sprinkle mixed berries, chopped nuts, and chia seeds on top.

2. Apple Cinnamon Oatmeal:

Ingredients:

- 1/2 cup rolled oats
- 1 cup water
- 1/2 apple, diced
- 1/2 teaspoon ground cinnamon
- 1 tablespoon chopped pecans

Instructions:

- Following package directions, Cook cooked rolled oats in water.
- Add diced apples, ground cinnamon and sprinkle chopped pecans.

3. Banana Nut Oatmeal:

Ingredients:

- 1/2 cup old-fashioned oats
- 1 cup water
- 1/2 banana, sliced

- 1 tablespoon almond butter
- 1 tablespoon chopped walnuts

Instructions:

- Follow the cooking directions on the pack of old-fashioned oats and cook them with water.
- Add sliced banana, almond butter, and sprinkle chopped walnuts on top.

4. Pumpkin Spice Oatmeal:

Ingredients:

- 1/2 cup steel-cut oats
- 1 cup water
- 2 tablespoons canned pumpkin puree
- 1/2 teaspoon pumpkin spice
- 1 tablespoon maple syrup (optional)

Instructions:

- Prepare steel-cuts porridge as instructed on its package.

- Add pumpkin paste, pumpkin powder and sweetening with maple sugar.

5. Chia Seed and Coconut Oatmeal:

Ingredients:

- 1/2 cup rolled oats
- 1 cup coconut milk (unsweetened)
- 1 tablespoon chia seeds
- 1/4 cup toasted coconut flakes

Instructions:

- Therefore, I cooked rolled oats in coconut milk as indicated on its packet.
- Add the chia seeds, then sprinkle the toasted coconut flake on top.

6. Chocolate Almond Oatmeal:

Ingredients:

- 1/2 cup old-fashioned oats
- 1 cup water
- 1 tablespoon unsweetened cocoa powder
- 1/2 banana, mashed

- 1 tablespoon almond butter

Instructions:

- Follow the directions on the package and cook old-fashioned oats in water.
- Mix in some cocoa powder, smashed bananas and almond butter.

7. Vanilla Peach Oatmeal:

Ingredients:

- 1/2 cup steel-cut oats
- 1 cup water
- 1/2 peach, diced
- 1/2 teaspoon vanilla extract
- 1 tablespoon slivered almonds

Instructions:

- Follow the instructions on a pack of steel-cut oats and cook in water.

- Add chopped peaches, vanilla extract, and sprinkle with sliced almonds on the top layer.

Go ahead and alter certain ingredients in order to make them more in line with what you enjoy eating and follow a healthier meal plan. The variations in Oatmeal can make breakfast sweet and healthy on The Pritikin Diet.

Certainly! The whole grains pancake that match with Pritikin plan are great and healthy.

Here's a simple recipe for whole grain pancakes for beginners:

Whole Grain Pancakes:

Ingredients:

- 1 cup whole wheat flour
- one half cup oat flour (you could make your own by grinding oats)
- 1 tablespoon ground flaxseeds
- 1 teaspoon baking powder
- 1/2 teaspoon baking soda
- 1/4 teaspoon salt
- 1/4 cup low-fat or fat free milk (or plant-based milk)
- One tablespoon of apple cider vinegar (or white vinegar)
- One big egg or a flaxseed egg, for egg-free option.

- One tablespoon of maple syrup or honey for flavor (optional)
- 1 teaspoon vanilla extract
- A bit of cooking spray or very small amount of oil.

Instructions:

1. **Prepare "Buttermilk":**
   - Mix the vinegar into the milk in a smaller bowl. For a couple of minutes, leave it to sour just a little bit. This creates a buttermilk substitute.

2. **Mix Dry Ingredients:**
   - Mix in a big bowl whole wheat flour, oat flour, ground flax seeds, sodium, baking powder sodium, and salt.

3. **Combine Wet Ingredients:**

   - Combine all the ingredients of "buttermilk" mixture, an egg (or egg made from flaxseeds), maple syrup or honey (only if you are going to use it) and vanilla extract in other separate bowl.

4. Combine Wet and Dry Ingredients:

- Mix in all of the wet ingredients with the dry ones, stirring it only till homogeneous. Ensure they do not get mixed too much; several lumps may be fine.

5. Preheat Pan:

- On medium heated non-stick griddle or skillet. Spray or lightly rub with oil.

6. Cook Pancakes:

- Pour a quarter cup of batter into the pre-heated griddle for each pancake. Turn up and cook the sides until they turn golden and are browned.

7. **Serve:**

- Addition of pure maple syrup, berries and sliced bananas can be served warm with these pancakes too.

8. **Optional Add-ins:**

- You could also add ½ cup of blueberries, finely chopped nuts, or a mushed ripe banana as options to the batter.

This is how this wholesome and filling breakfast was made of whole grain pancakes. Try out various whole grains and toppings based on your dietary preferences, provided they align with Pritikin diet principles.

Involves the use of nutritious ingredients with reduced additional sugar, oil, and oil in a bid to make delicious Pritkini scramble and omelet.

Here are a couple of recipes to get you started:

1. Vegetable Scramble:

Ingredients:

- 1 teaspoon olive oil
- 1/4 cup diced onion
- 1/4 cup diced bell peppers of various colors.
- 1/4 cup diced zucchini
- 1/4 cup cherry tomatoes, halved
- To eggs (or egg whites) two whole.
- Salt and pepper to taste

For garnish, fresh herbs e.g., parsley, chives.

Instructions:

Sauté Vegetables:

- Put olive oil into a frying pan and place it on a hot plate. Then add onions, bell peppers, and zucchinis Sauté until vegetables are tender.

Add Tomatoes:

- Cook for one to two minutes while adding cherry tomatoes to soften them as well.

Scramble Eggs:

- Place some vegetables aside, pour the beaten eggs in. Just let the eggs relax a little and then scramble them together with the veggies.

Season:

- Sprinkle some salt and pepper into it depending on your preference.

Garnish:

- Serve garnished with herbs, such as parsley or chives.

2. Spinach and Mushroom Omelet:

Ingredients:

- 1 teaspoon olive oil
- 1/4 cup sliced mushrooms
- 1 cup fresh spinach
- Two big eggs or egg whites.
- Salt and pepper to taste
- Optional: A little bit of feta-cheese, 1 tablespoon.

Instructions:

Sauté Mushrooms:

- Put in olive oil in a nonstick pan on the stove top using medium heat. mushroom slices until they become juicy.

Add Spinach:

- Wilt the spinach in a fresh skillet.

Prepare Eggs:

- In a bowl, mix the eggs. Put the eggs on top of the mushrooms and spinach.

Cook Omelet:

- Place the eggs on the sides to let them set there. Use a spatula to raise the omelet sides for some raw egg juice to drip under.

Season and Add Cheese (Optional):

- Season with salt and pepper. Add a little feta cheese on top of one-half of an omelet if possible.

Fold and Serve:

- After the eggs are completely cooked, fold the omelet and place it on your plate.

You may also substitute some of the ingredients in these recipes with items that are approved by the Pritikin program including diced tomatoes, onions and herbs. Include extra fats in your diet but make sure it is low on saturated and use frying technique that involve little amount of oil or cookware made without stickiness. Omelets and scrambles make for the tastiest breakfasts, which meet the dietary needs of the Pritikin Eating plan.

CHAPTER 4

LUNCH IDEALS

Whole foods in their natural state can also fill you up without all those calories, make for the best lunch in a Pritikin diet plan.

Here are some lunch ideas for beginners following the Pritikin Diet:

1. Grilled Chicken Salad:

- Chicken breast grills, over mixed greens (spinach, arugula, romaine), cherry tomatoes, cucumbers, and light vinaigrette.

2. Quinoa and Vegetable Bowl:

- Quinoa sautéed with different colored vegetables (peppers, zucchini, cherry tomato), dressed with a lemon-tahini sauce. Top with chopped fresh herbs.

3. Black Bean and Avocado Wrap:

- Burrito bowl including whole wheat or sprouted grain wrap and having black beans,
- diced avocado, salsa, shredded lettuce, squeezes of lime.

4 Salmon and Vegetable Stir-Fry:

- A stir-fry of salmon with broccoli, snow peas, carrots, and sweet red bell peppers. Serve on brown rice or cauliflower rice.

5. Mediterranean Chickpea Salad:

- Cherry tomatoes, cucumbers, red onions, Kalamata, and feta with chickpeas. Use olive oil with some lemon juice and herbs.

6. Sweet Potato and Lentil Soup:

- Sweet potato and lentil soup that can be enriched with other greens such as kale or spinach. Add flavors like herbs and spices.

7. Turkey and Veggie Lettuce Wraps:

- Stir fry lean ground turmeric, diced pepper, onion, chilies, chives and oregano. Wrap it into large lettuce leaves for serve.

8. Whole Grain Pasta with Pesto and Vegetables:

- Whole grain pasta and pesto made with basil, cherry tomatoes, and broccoli. Sprinkle with pine nuts.

9. Greek Salad with Grilled Shrimp:

Shrimps grilled on a bed of mixed lettuce, with cherry tomatoes, cucumber, red onion, feta cheese and light dressing of Greek.

10. Vegetarian Buddha Bowl:

- For example, sweet potatoes roasted in brown rice or quinoa tossed with sautéed kale, avocado slices, and tahini dressing drizzled on top.

11. Eggplant and Chickpea Curry:

- Chickpeas and eggplant curry with onions and tomatoes combined with various spices. Serving the dish over gluten free rice option such as brown rice or cauliflower can make the meal even healthier.

12. Tuna and White Bean Salad:

- Tuna with white beans, cherry tomatoes, red onion, and fresh herbs. Dress in olive oil and lemon juice.

13. Caprice Stuffed Portobello Mushrooms:

- Fresh mozzarella, basil, and tomato slices inside Portobello mushrooms. Drizzle with balsamic glaze.

14. Asian-Inspired Tofu Stir-Fry:

- Tofu stir fried with colorful vegetables (broccoli, bell pepper, and snow peas served on the side dipped in a light soy and ginger sauce. Serve over brown rice.

15. Chicken and Vegetable Skewers:

- For example, grilled chicken and vegetable skewers served alongside quinoa or brown rice. Apply a citrus-herb vinaigrette.

Do not forget to include a range from vegetables, lean protein, whole grains and healthy fat to your lunchtime meal's Consider your calorie burn rate and adjust your portion size to suit, if need be. Drinking enough water and herbal tea is equally important. Customize these for your tastes and have an enjoyable, fulfilling lunch on Pitkin's diet.

Whole and unprocessed food can be both satisfying and also provide a nutritious lunch when following the Pritikin Diet.

Here are some lunch ideas for beginners following the Pritikin Diet:

1. Grilled Chicken Salad:

- Grilled chicken breast slices on a bed of mixed greens (spinach, arugula, and romaine) with cherry tomatoes, cucumber, and light vinaigrette dressing.

2. Quinoa and Vegetable Bowl:

- Sautéed quinoa with colorful vegetables (bell pepper, zucchini, and cherry tomato) and finished with tahini vinaigrette. Top with chopped fresh herbs.

3. Black Bean and Avocado Wrap:

- Sandwich made using whole wheat or sprouted grains stuffed with black beans, chopped avocado, salsa, shredded lettuce, and squirted lime juice.

4. Salmon and Vegetable Stir-Fry:

- Stir frying salmon with broccoli, snow peas, carrot, and red pepper. Serve over brown or cauliflower rice.

5. Mediterranean Chickpea Salad:

- A mixture of chickpeas and fresh cherry tomatoes, cucumber, red onion, Kalamata olives, feta cheese. The recipe for dressing should involve using olive oil, lemon juice among other herbs.

6. Sweet Potato and Lentil Soup:

- Homemade sweet potato and lentil soup including some vegetables such as kale or spinach can be eaten by pregnant women. Add a little bit of flavor using herbs and spices.

7. Turkey and Veggie Lettuce Wraps:

- Diced bell peppers, onion, and spice marinated lean ground turkey. Layer mixture inside large lettuce leaves to make it into wraps.

8. Whole Grain Pasta with Pesto and Vegetables:

- Pasta whole grain tossed in homemade basil pesto with tomato cherries and broccoli steaming. Sprinkle with pine nuts.

9. Greek Salad with Grilled Shrimp:

- Grilled shrimp over mixed greens and tomato with cucumber, red onion, feta cheese, and Greek dressing.

10. Vegetarian Buddha Bowl:

- Ingredients: Quinoa (cooked), cherry tomatoes, cucumbers, red onion, feta,

Kalamata olives. Drizzle with olive oil and lemon sauce.

11. Salmon and Asparagus Salad:

- **Ingredients**: Salmon (grilled or baked), asparagus spears, mixed greens, cherry Salad, dressed with a lemon-dill vinaigrette.

12. Pesto Chicken Salad:

Ingredients: Chicken, salad mix, cherry tomatoes, and pine nuts. Wearing a pesto pitted on a pirtikin basis.

13. Southwest Black Bean Salad:

- **Ingredients**: Black beans with corn, cherry tomatoes, red onion, and cilantro. Vinaigrette de lime-cumin.

14. Roasted Beet and Goat Cheese Salad:

- Ingredients: Beetroot roasted, mixed greens, goat cheese and walnut. Sautéed vinegar dressing is great for balsamic

vinegar topped dressings with just
enough olive oil.

15. Avocado and Chickpea Salad:

- Ingredients: Avocado dressing chickpea, cherry tomato, cucumber and red onion. Salad dressing made of lime and cilantro.

Also make sure you pay attention to portions and avoid fatty meats in your salad while opting for lean protein options with lots of colorful veggies and healthy fats. Be bold enough to mix up new ingredients or different styles of dressing while still following the Pritikin Diet guidelines.

Certainly! The Pritikin diet allows one to consume mouthwatering plant-based sandwiches and burgers.

Here are some ideas for beginners:

Plant-Based Sandwiches:

1. **Hummus and Veggie Sandwich:**
   - Cover whole wheat bread with hummus. Add sliced cucumbers, tomatoes, red onions, and shredded romaine lettuce.

2. **Avocado and Black Bean Wrap**:
   - Spread mashed avocado on a whole wheat or sprouted grain tortilla and top with black beans, diced tomatoes, corn, and a sprinkling of cilantro.

3. **Chickpea Salad Sandwich:**
   - Smashed chickpeas with the avocado, with some diced celery, red onions, and a squirt of lemon juice therein. Whole grain bread with lettuce, and tomato

4. **Peanut Butter and Banana Sandwich:**

- Take whole grain bread spread with natural peanut butter layered with sliced bananas on it. One can also make it more special by adding some drops of honey.

5. **Mushroom and Spinach Panini:**
   - Cook the mushrooms and spinach with garlic. Lays on two slices of whole-grain bread for about five minutes in the panini maker.

6. **Eggplant and Hummus Wrap:**
   - Sautéed eggplant, hummus spread wrap, fresh spinach & tomatoes.

7. **Mango and Black Bean Quesadilla:**
   - Stuff a whole wheat tortilla with black beans, mango in dice form, red onion, and a pinch of cumin. Wrap up and cook in a skillet, making them crispy

8. **Tofu and Vegetable:**
   - Dip tofu in soy-ginger marinade and place it onto whole grain bagel with pickled veggies, cucumbers and coriander.

9. **Black Bean and Quinoa Burger:**
   - Mash black beans and mix this with cooked quinoa, chopped onion, and add herbs and spices. Shape it into patties then roast or bake them. Serve on whole grain buns.

10. **Sweet Potato and Lentil Burger:**
   - Mix and mash together cooked sweet potatoes, mashed lentils, and breadcrumbs. Mound into patties, bake or fry them in pan. Add to lettuce wraps or whole grain buns.

11. **Chickpea and Spinach Burger:**
   - Chickpeas, spinach, and spice should be blended using a food processer. Form into patties and cook. Top with your favorite toppings and serve on whole grain bun.

12. **Portobello Mushroom Burger**:

- The Portobello mushroom caps can be grilled or roasted and served as a burger along with some lettuce, tomatoes and half-avocado.

13. **Quinoa and Black-Eyed Pea Burger**:

- Blend cooked grains of quinoa, mash black-eyed peas, dice bell pepper and add all required seasonings. Shape into patties and cook. Serve on whole grain buns.

14. **Falafel Burger**:

- Using chickpeas mixed with herbs and spices and form into patties." Serve in a whole grain pita with lettuce, tomato, and tahini dressing.

15. **Spicy Lentil Burger**:

- Mix cooked lentils with breadcrumbs, chopped jalapeños, and spices. Form into patties and cook. Serve on whole grain buns.

16. **Soy and Vegetable Burger**:

- Incorporate sautéed vegetables and TVP with soy sauce and preferably a spice of your choice. Shape into patties and cook. Serve on

17. **whole grain buns.**
    - Ensure you have lots of fresh vegetables and whole grain in your plant-based sandwiches and burger. As long as you follow the fundamental principles, have fun with different flavors, and toppings until you are satisfied.

CHAPTER 5

DINNER DELIGHTS

Pritikin's diet has a very strict policy in terms of creating savory and healthy dinners. This policy includes a number of unprocessed foods.

Here are some dinner ideas for beginners:

1. Grilled Salmon with Lemon-Dill Sauce:

- Lightly grilled salmon fillet with lemon-dill sauce. Serve it with steamed broccoli and quinoa.

2. Vegetable Stir-Fry with Tofu:

- Tofu mixed together with different colored foods like broccoli, snaps, and bell pepper as an accompaniment in a light ginger/soy sauce. Serve over brown rice.

3. Baked Chicken Breast with Roasted Vegetables:

- A baked chicken breast seasoned with herbs, along with a side of roasted sweet potatoes, carrots and Brussels' sprout.

4. Chickpea and Spinach Curry:

- Tasty curry prepared using tomatoes, onions, and spices and chickpeas, and spinach. Serve over brown rice.

5. Pasta Primavera with Grilled Chicken:

- Pasta made from whole grain tossed with different roasted veggies and grilled chicken piece. A tomato based sauce or a light oil dressing.

6. Turkey and Quinoa Stuffed Peppers:

- Prepared ground turkey seasoned with quinoa, black beans, corn, spices, stuffed inside bell peppers, and baked.

7. Mushroom and Lentil Stew:

- Stew of mushrooms and lentils with carrots, celery, as well as onions. You can also opt to season it with herbs such as thyme and rosemary.

8. Shrimp and Vegetable Skewers:

- Shrimps and vegetables grilled with fresh herbs and lemon. Offer with quinoa as a side dish or green salad.

9. Eggplant Parmesan:

- Part-skim mozzarella on top of baked eggplant strips mixed with marinara sauce. Serve over whole wheat pasta.

10. Cauliflower and Chickpea Tacos:

- Cauliflower and chickpeas roasted in taco spiced, whole grain tortillas with lettuce, tomatoes, and salsa.

11. Soy-Ginger Glazed Cod:

- Glazed with a soy-ginger sauce and baked or oven roasted cod fillets". Serve with steamed bok Choy or rice.

12. Quinoa and Black Bean Bowl:

- Black beans blended with quinoa, corn, diced tomatoes and avocado. Lime-cumin vinaigrette on top.

13. Stir-Fried Tofu and Broccoli:

- A light garlic and soy stir fry of tofu and broccoli. Serve over cauliflower rice.

14. Lemon Herb Chicken with Asparagus:

- Broiled chicken breast with lemon and herb seasoning, accompanied by roasted asparagus.

15. Sweet Potato and Lentil Shepherd's Pie:

- Savory tomato sauce with lentils and vegetables, baked mashed sweet potatoes on top and get out the fork.

Ensure that you have included many different types of vegetables, lean proteins and wholegrain products in your dinnertimes. Make sure adjust your portions depending on your needs, activity levels, etc. Water and herbal teas should also be used to keep one's body hydrated. Please note that you can make adjustments within these ideas based on your preference and satisfy hunger while maintaining health when doing it the Pritikin way.

LEAN PROTEIN ENTRESS

Absolutely! The diet calls for you to have lean protein in every meal.

Here are some ideas for lean protein entrees for beginners:

1. Grilled Chicken Breast:

- Salted season chicken breasts should be grilled until it is ready for consumption. Serve it with steamed vegetables or mixed greens.

2. Baked Salmon:

- Marinate season salmon with lemon, dill, and little bit oil. Let the salmon flake. Combine with roasted candied yams and broccoli.

3. Turkey and Vegetable Stir-Fry:

- Sauté lean ground turkey with a medley of vibrant veggies (pepper, green beans, corn) and a gentle soy-based ginger sauce. Serve over brown rice.

4. Vegetarian Chili with Black Beans:

- Go for a hearty chili with black beans, tomatoes, onions, and spices. Sprinkle with chopped green onions and a spoonful of Greek yoghurt.

5. Grilled Shrimp Skewers:

- Place the shrimps in a marinade of lemon, garlic, and herbs. Thread onto skewers and grill. With a plate of steamed asparagus and quinoa on the side.

6. Lemon Herb Baked Cod:

- Coat seasoned cod fillets with some drops of olive oil, lemons, and herbs.

Bake for about 10 minutes until the fish is done flaking. Serve with a quinoa salad.

7. Lentil and Vegetable Curry:

- Add to it cooked lentils along with many vegetables simmered in a tasty curry
- based on tomatoes, onion, and spices. Serve over cauliflower rice.

8. Tofu and Broccoli Stir-Fry:

- Cook tofu with broccoli in a light garlic and soy sauce. Alternatively, serve it on a bed of brown rice or try it served hot over quinoa.

9. Chicken and Vegetable Kebabs:

- Colorful bell peppers, cherry tomatoes, and onions can be skewered together with colorful chicken breast chunks and grilled afterward. Serve with couscous as a side dish.

10. Quinoa and Black Bean Stuffed Peppers:

- Stuff in bell peppers a mixture of cooked quinoa and black beans, diced vegetables. Bake until peppers are tender.

11. Egg White Omelet with Vegetables:

- Use egg whites and cook veggies such as spinach, bell peppers, and tomatoes to make an omelet.

12. Turkey and Quinoa Meatballs:

- Combine ground turkey breast meat fried in olive oil with quinoa flakes, chopped onion, and basil or oregano spices. Form into meatballs and bake. Serve with a tomato sauce.

13. Chickpea and Spinach Sauté:

- Pan-fry some chickpeas, garlic, cherry tomatoes, and spinach. Sprinkle with herbs and lay over whole wheat Couscous.
- Stir-fry chickpeas, spinach and whole garlic pods together with cherry

tomatoes. Add herbs, and garnish over a bed of whole wheat couscous.

4. Grilled Chicken Salad:

- Cherry tomato, cucumber salad with a side of grilled chicken breast and mixed greens garnished with a light vinaigrette dressing.

15. Soy-Ginger Glazed Tofu:

- Tofu marinated in tofu-soy ginger glaze and baked or grilled till golden. Serve alongside steamed broccoli and brown rice.

Make sure to control the portion sizes as well as select a healthier method of cooking. The Pritikin Diet emphasizes lean protein entrees with different tastes and nutrients suitable for such meal. Make these adjustments to match with what you prefer, you can eat that full meal in balance.

Homemade sauce and dressing is an alternative of adding flavor to your meals as per Pritkin's principles.

Here are some simple and Pritikin-friendly recipes for sauces and dressings:

1. Homemade Sauces:

- Tomato Basil Marinara:

Ingredients:

- crushed tomatoes with no added sugar in one can (28 oz.)
- 2 cloves garlic, minced
- 1 tablespoon olive oil
- 1 teaspoon dried basil
- Salt and pepper to taste

Instructions:

- Put minced garlic into a saucepan and simmer it in olive oil until its fragrance comes off.

- Put in some canned tomatoes as well as basil. Cook covered at a low flame for fifteen to twenty minutes, stirring every now and then.
- Sprinkle with salt and black pepper at convenience.

3. Lemon Herb Vinaigrette:

Ingredients:

- 1/4 cup fresh lemon juice
- 2 tablespoons extra-virgin olive oil
- 1 teaspoon Dijon mustard
- 1 clove garlic, minced
- One teaspoon of any dried herb (e.g., oregano, thyme, or basil).

4. Salt and pepper to taste

Instructions:

- Mix together lemon juice, olive oil, Dijon mustard, garlic, and herbs.
- Sprinkle seasoning with salt and pepper.

4. Soy-Ginger Glaze:

Ingredients:

- A fourth cup of low sodium soya sauce
- 1 tablespoon rice vinegar
- 1 tablespoon fresh ginger, grated
- 1 clove garlic, minced
- One tablespoon of honey if you want it to be a little sweeter

Instructions:

- Mix soy sauce, rice vinegar, grated ginger, minced garlic and honey in a bowl.

5. Creamy Avocado Sauce:

Ingredients:

- 1 ripe avocado
- Two tablespoons plain Greek yogurt or fat free.
- 1 tablespoon lime juice
- 1 clove garlic, minced
- Salt and pepper to taste

Instructions:

- Squish the ready for eating avocado and mix it with the Greek yogurt, lime juice, mingled garlic, salt and pepper.

Homemade Dressings:

1. Balsamic Vinaigrette

Ingredients:

- 3 tablespoons balsamic vinegar
- 2 tablespoons extra-virgin olive oil
- 1 teaspoon Dijon mustard
- A teaspoon of honey is optional as a sweetener.
- Salt and pepper to taste

Instructions:

- Mix balsamic vinegar, olive oil, Dijon mustard and honey if you would like.
- Add salt and pepper for seasoning.

2. Tahini-Lemon Dressing:

Ingredients:

- 2 tablespoons tahini
- 2 tablespoons fresh lemon juice
- 1 clove garlic, minced
- As per consistency, one may use a tablespoon of water (more is optional).
- Salt and pepper to taste

Instructions:

- Combine together tahini, lemon juice, chopped garlic, and some water to create a homogeneous mixture.
- Dust with salt and pepper to taste.

3. Herbed Greek Yogurt Dressing:

Ingredients:

- half a cup of fat free Greek plain yogurt
- 2 tablespoons fresh lemon juice

- 1 tablespoon of fresh herbs (dill, parsley, and chives).
- Salt and pepper to taste

Instructions:

- Combine Greek yogurt with lemon juice and fresh chopped herbs.
- Add seasoning as per taste using salt and pepper.

4. Cilantro-Lime Dressing:

Ingredients:

- 1/4 cup fresh lime juice
- 2 tablespoons chopped fresh cilantro
- 1 tablespoon olive oil
- 1 teaspoon honey (can be added for sweetness).
- Salt and pepper to taste

Instructions:

- Mix lime juice, chopped cilantro, olive oil and honey (optional) in a bowl.

- Add salt and pepper to your liking, seasoned to taste.

Please feel free to tweak those recipes for your own preferences. Such homemade sauces and dressing are healthy alternatives that will bring some zest into your food but still be suitable for someone following Pritikin diet program.

CHAPTER 6

SNACKS AND APPETIZERS

Certainly! Taking healthy snacks and appetizers as part of your Pritikin diet will keep you satiate until the next meal.

Here are some ideas for snacks and appetizers for beginners:

Healthy Snacks:

1. **Fresh Fruit:**
   - Get some fresh fruit for dessert in form of cut apples, berries, orange slices, and bananas.

2. **Vegetable Sticks with Hummus:**
   - Use a healthy dip with some sticks of cut up carrots, cucumbers, or bell peppers.

3. **Greek Yogurt with Berries:**
   - Opt for plain non-fat Greek yogurt with fresh berries and a touch of honey.

4. Nuts and Seeds Mix:

- Mix unroasted almonds, walnut nuts and pumpkin seeds into a healthier snacks alternative.

5. Whole Grain Crackers with Guacamole:

- The crackers can also be paired with a homemade guacamole made from mashed avocado, lime juice, and diced tomato.

6. Hard-Boiled Eggs:

- Make hard-boiled eggs for a quick-snack that is packed in proteins.

7. Cherry Tomatoes with Mozzarella:

- Spread top whole grain baguette slices with mixture of diced avocado, tomato, garlic, and basil.

8. Roasted Chickpeas:

- Make crispy healthy roast chickpeas with some drizzled virgin olive oil, seasoning spices and herbs, if you want crispy healthy roast snack.

9. Quinoa Salad Cups:

- A great light appetizer would be to spoon quinoa salad into endive or lettuce cups.

10. Cucumber Roll-Ups:

- Use cucumber slices as wrappings for a low-carb and high-protein appetizer.

11. Artichoke and Spinach Dip (Lightened):

- Opt for a healthier variant, artichoke and spinach dip with Greek yogurt and light cream cheese. Serve with vegetable sticks.

The snacks and appetizers ensure that there is a combination of nutrients but not contradicting the Pritikin diet. Portion sizes should be modified in accordance with people. Play around to determine which Pritikin-friendly snack you prefer best.

NUTRIENT PACKED SNACK IDEAS

The snacks that one can have while doing the Pritikin diet are delicious and healthy as well.

Here are some nutrient-packed snack ideas that align with the principles of the Pritikin Diet:

1. **Fresh Fruit with Almond Butter:**
   - Half an apple sliced, pear, banana, and The mixture of fiber, vitamins, and healthful fat offers an excellent balance.

2. **Vegetable Sticks with Hummus:**
   - A small number of carrot sticks, cucumber slices, and bell pepper strips along with an equivalent portion of homemade or market-ready low fat humors.

3. **Greek Yogurt Parfait:**
   - A layer of non-fat Greek yogurt on top of berry mix (blueberries, strawberries and

raspberries), nut sprinkles such as almonds and walnuts and then some honey on top.

4. Edamame:

- Edamame steamed with a few grains of salt. They have high levels of edamame as a plant protein and fiber.

5. Mixed Nuts and Seeds:

- Few pieces of raw, non-salted nuts and seeds, for example, almonds, walnuts, and pumpkin seeds. This includes the good fats as well as vital nutrients.

6. Whole Grain Crackers with Avocado:

- Avocado spread on whole grain or multigrain crackers. Avocado provides high levels of mono-unsaturated fats and fiber.

7. Homemade Trail Mix:

- Combine raw nuts, seeds, and dried fruits. Use unsweetened dried fruits only without any sugary ingredients.

8. **Cottage Cheese with Pineapple**:
   - Fresh cut up pineapple on a low-fat cottage cheese serving. Pineapple also combines well with cottage cheese, which contains proteins.

9. **Cherry Tomatoes with Balsamic Glaze:**
   - A balsamic drizzle over cherry tomatoes. It is a calorie friendly snack that has high level of antioxidants.

10. **Roasted Chickpeas:**
   - Toast some freshly roasted chickpeas in a pan, adding your preferred seasoning or spices.

11. **Seaweed Snacks:**
   - The seaweed snack is low calorie, but high in minerals. Consequently, they can be enjoyed as a sweet treat.

12. **Frozen Grapes:**
   - Frozen grapes are an excellent treat and can be eaten as fruit as well. They constitute a healthy substitute for sweet frozen items.

Make sure you control the size of your plates by practicing portion control, and also listen to the signals from your stomach that indicate whether or not you are hungry. Additionally, avoid packaged snack that contain unnecessary amount of sugar and salt. It is important that you ask for guidance from a health care provider or nutritionist when planning drastic dietary changes.

CHAPTER 7

DESSERTS AND TREATS

It might be difficult to prepare desserts and other sweet things when following the Pritikin Diet, which restricts the intake of sugar additions and emphasizes on natural, unrefined meals. Nevertheless, you can also indulge in other naturally sweet snacks.

Here are a few ideas:

1. **Baked Apples:**
- Make a hole in the middle of an apple and stuff it with cinnamon and a few pieces of nuts. Allow the fruit to become tender by baking. Use non-fat Greek yoghurt to garnish it.

2. **Berries with Mint:**
- Crush ripe berries such as strawberries, blueberries, and raspberries. Top up with some fresh mint leaves for a fresher, natural after-dessert taste.

3. Grilled Pineapple:

- Prepare fresh slices of pineapple while it is on the grill until caramelization occurs. Natural sugars found in the pineapple increase, making it even more delicious.

4. Fruit Salad with Citrus Dressing:

- Mix different types of fruits such as melons, citrus segments, kiwi or other fruit varieties. Add flair by tossing it with a dressing made of fresh orange or grapefruit juice.

5. Chia Seed Pudding:

- Stir in non-fat milk or almond milk using chia seeds. Refrigerate for it to become thick. Add some fresh berry fruits on top for nutrition full and delicious pudding.

6. Frozen Banana Bites:

- Cut small bites of banana in to it, then dunk them into melted dark chocolate (with minimum 70% Cocoa. Freeze until the chocolate hardens.

7. Yogurt Parfait:

* Add some texture by layering non-fat Greek yogurt with fresh fruit and chopped nuts or seeds.

8. Date and Nut Balls:

* Combine dates and nuts like almonds or walnut using a food processor. Making small balls is the way of going about it for a sweeter, nuttier treat.

9. Baked Pears with Cinnamon:

* Cut off pear slices and dust them with cinnamon. Place in an oven and bake until pear is tender. Serve warm for an indulging dessert.

10.   Coconut and Berry Sorbet:

- Mix frozen berries and coconut water together in a blender till it becomes smooth. To make sorbet, freeze mixture to obtain a cool one.

11.   Mango Sorbet:

- Mash ripe mangoes, chill them. This is a straightforward and naturally sweet frozen treat.

12.   Homemade Fruit Sorbet:

- Combine frozen fruits such as berries, mangoes or pineapples with some water or fruit juice for a DIY sorbet.

Ensure you stick to smaller portions when choosing desserts and always pick those compliant with the Pritikin diet principle involving whole, unprocessed foods. You should seek medical advice or consult with a nutritionist if you want to make substantial modifications in your diet.

SWEET ENDING WITH A HEALTHY TWIST

Certainly! Here's a sweet ending with a healthy twist for those following the Pritikin Diet:

1. **Chocolate Avocado Mousse:**
- 2 ripe avocados
- 1/4 cup unsweetened cocoa powder
- 1/4 cup low fat Greek yogurt.
- 1/4 cup of pure maple syrup or honey
- 1 teaspoon vanilla extract
- A pinch of salt

Instructions:

- Remove the peels and pits of the avocado and put it in the blender.
- Make sure to mix cocoa powder, Greek yogurt, maple syrup or honey with some additional ingredients such as vanilla extract and a pinch of salt.
- Mix it well together, using a stick blender or food processor, and occasionally scrape

down the sides to blend any pieces that may have become stuck on them.

- Try out different tastes and add more maple syrup or honey until desired sweetness is achieved.
- Refrigerate it for at least thirty minutes prior to serving.
- Smaller bowls or glass serve it. Garnish with fresh berries/chopped nuts.
- Healthier chocolate avocado mousse that is just as indulgent as "regular" chocolate mousse. The avocados contribute to creaminess as well as some healthy fats, whilst Greek yoghurt brings in the additional protein content. There are natural sweet ingredients such as maple syrup or honey, which serve best instead of refined sugar in satisfying the sweet craving.

Ensure that you also take sweeteners, but not too much, and find ways of putting whole foods into it. Ensure that you discuss any significant changes in your diet with a healthcare provider, consultant, and/or nutritionist prior taking any action.

FRUIT BASED DESSERTS

There is no doubt that fruit-based deserts will be fantastic choices for people on the Pritikin diet because they are naturally sweet and have fibers and vitamins.

 Here are some delicious fruit-based dessert ideas:

1. **Grilled Fruit Skewers:**
- Thread cubes of pineapples, mangoes and strawberries. Grill until they caramelize slightly. Drizzle some balsamic glaze over it and serve as well.

2. **Mixed Berry Parfait:**
- Use sliced or quartered, fresh berries (strawberries, blueberries, raspberries) layered between spoonful of non-fat Greek yogurt and a sprinkling of chopped nuts or seeds.

3. **Fruit Salad with Citrus Mint Dressing:**
- Mix different kinds of crisp fruits such as melons, berries, and citruses. Toss in a dressing using freshly squeezed orange juice, and chopped mint.

4. **Stuffed Baked Apples:**
- Stuff some core apples with a mixture of chopped nuts, raisins and dusted cinnamon. Bake until apples soften well.

5. **Peach Melba:**
- Freshly cut top peaches sprinkled with some raspberries, drizzled on by honey, and placed on top of small scoop of nonfat Greek yogurt. Drizzle it all over with a wee bit of honey.

6. **Frozen Banana "Ice Cream":**

- Mix frozen ripe bananas into a smooth consistency. You can always opt for a dash of almond milk while adding it. Top it off with finely chopped nuts, berries, and even cinnamon.

7. **Berry Sorbet:**
- Mix some frozen berry with a little water or juice without sugar and make it smooth. Let it sit in the fridge for some hours and then serve chilled.

8. **Mango Salsa:**
- Chop fresh mango into small pieces, add chopped mint, lime juice, and a pinch of red chili powder. Eat it alone or with one-whole grain tortilla chips.

9. **Fruit Kabobs with Yogurt Dip:**
- Put various small fruit pieces on skewers. Serve next to a small bowl of non-fat Greek yogurt for dipping.

10.   **Orange and Kiwi Salad:**

- For a healthy citrus salad, mix sliced oranges with kiwi. Drizzle lightly with honey; garnish with fresh mint.

11.   **Frozen Grapes**:
- For a fun, sweet, and cold snack eat frozen grapes. It is very easy making such desserts.

12.   **Berry Popsicles:**
- Prepare a pureed fruit mix using berries then pour it in popsicle molds. Make freeze for a delicious sugar free and homemade popsicle.

While these fruit-based desserts are sweet and irresistible, they comprise of vitamins, antioxidants and natural content. Feel free to consume them as per a normal but Pritikin diet.

Never undertake dramatic changes in your diet without involving a healthcare provider or a nutritionist.

CHAPTER 8

MEAL PLANNING AND PREPPING

It is important for someone trying to follow the Pritikin Diet to plan meals and prepare them ahead of time to make sure that they have healthy snacks at hand whenever they get hungry.

Here's a guide to help beginners with meal planning and prepping for the Pritikin Diet:

1. Understand Pritikin Diet Principles:

- Focus on whole foods: Pick natural or whole foods such as fruits, vegetables, whole grains, lean meats, and beans.

Limit saturated fats and cholesterol: Choose lean proteins like fish, chicken and a vegetable basis.

Minimize added sugars and salt: Use natural sweets for the taste and flavor food by herbs and spices except the salt.

2. Create a Weekly Meal Plan:
- Breakfast:
- Oatmeal with fresh fruits and nuts.
- Greek yogurt parfait with berries.
- Scrambled eggs with vegetables.

3 **Lunch:**

- Salad with grilled chicken or tofu and vegetables.
- Mixed bowl of quinoa or brown rice along with vegetables.
- Whole grain bean/ lentil soup.

5. Dinner:

- They suggest baked white fish or skinless chicken breast with steamed vegetables.
- Tofu or tempeh stir fry with rainbow vegetables.
- Turkey chili with bean and tomato.

   6. Snacks:

- An apple or two together with some nuts.
- Vegetable sticks with hummus.
- Greek yogurt and honey drizzle.

6. Plan for Variety:

- Ensure that you eat a lot of different kind of foods like fruits, vegetables, whole grains, and proteins to get different nutrients.
- Change your style of cooking in order not to bore yourself. For example, try roast, steam or grill.

7. Batch Cooking:

- Roast all grains in bulk as well as a few other types of protein at the start of the week.
- Make it easy to prepare meals by breaking down meal portions into smaller containers and storing them individually.

8. Prep Vegetables and Fruits:

- Prepare fruits and veggies into bite-size pieces for snacks or to add in a salad.
- Cut up vegetables are more convenient for cooking a stir-fry, to add them in an omelette or as a side.

9. Protein Preparation:

- Cooking batches of chicken, fish, or tofu throughout the week on the grill or oven.
- Make sure that a portion of it is frozen and put aside for later portions.

10. Make Healthy Sauces and Dressings:

- To boost flavor without compromising health, prepare homemade, Pritikin-friendly sauces and dressings beforehand.

11. Stock Healthy Staples:

- Always ensure that you have a supply of whole grains, beans, canned tomatoes, low-salt broth, and healthy snacks in your pantry.

12. Portion Control:

- Provided with small, portioned container this will go a long way in avoiding overindulgence.

10. Stay Hydrated:

- Always drink a lot of water during the day in order to keep well hydrated.

11. Be Flexible:

- Build a flexible plan. Tailor your food and your meals to suit your tastes, your seasonal produce, and your schedule.

12. Monitor Progress:

- Maintain a journal of your meals, paying attention to how each type of food affects you.

Remember, consistency is key. This makes it easier for you to plan for meals and prepare the required food on the Pritikin Diet. One should always seek the opinion of a healthcare specialist or the nutritionist, for individual suggestions or recommendations.

It also entails having a weekly menu that comprises of lots of fresh and unadulterated products with essential nutrients.

Here's a sample weekly meal plan for beginners:

Day 1:

Breakfast:

- Fresh berries mixed with oatmeal served together with some chopped nuts.

- Green tea or black coffee.

Lunch:

- Mixed greens, cherry tomatoes, cucumber grilled chicken salad with a balsamic and dijon dressing.

Dinner:

- Salmon bake with lemon and herbs. temperature: °C
- Steamed broccoli, carrots, and quinoa pilaf.
- Mixed fruit salad for dessert.

Day 2:

Breakfast:

- Poached egg on whole grain toast with avacado slices.
- Herbal tea or black coffee.

Lunch:

- Lentil and vegetable soup.
- Whole grain roll or bread.

Dinner:

- Stir-fry tofu with multicolor vegetable mix.
- Brown rice.
- Sliced mango for dessert.

Day 3:

Breakfast:

- Parfait composed of various layers of crisp grains, mixed berry fruit topping, and Greek style yogurt.
- Green tea or black coffee.

Lunch:

- Whole-wheat tortillas filled with turkey and vegetables.

- Light mixed green salad served with vinaigrette.

Dinner:

- Quinoa and grilled shrimp skewers.
- Roasted Brussels sprouts and asparagus.
- Dessert: baked apple with cinnamon.

Day 4:

Breakfast:

- Spinach smoothie with banana, berry, almond milk.
- Herbal tea or black coffee.

Lunch:

- Chicken curry and rice, or chickpeas and vegetable curry with brown rice.

Dinner:

- Tomato-Basil-topped baked chicken breast.
- Sweet potato wedges.
- Fresh fruit salad for dessert.

Day 5:

Breakfast:

- Sautéed spinach, scrambled eggs with tomatoes.
- Green tea or black coffee.

Lunch:

- Mixed vegetables quinoa salad with a tahini-lemon dressing.

Dinner:

- Freshly grilled cod fillet accompanied with some fresh lemon juice.
- Steamed broccoli and cauliflower.
- For desserts, we had frozen banana slices with a drizzle of dark chocolate.

Day 6:

Breakfast:

- Strawberry-topped whole grain pancakes with Greek yogurt.
- Herbal tea or black coffee.

Lunch:

- Mozzarella, basil, and tomato Capers salad.
- Whole grain crackers.

Dinner:

- Zucchini noodles with Turkey Meatballs Bake.
- Roasted bell peppers.
- Mixed berries for dessert.

Day 7:

Breakfast:

- Almond milk chia seed pudding with fresh mango slices on top.
- Green tea or black coffee.

Lunch:

- Black bean, quinoa bowl with salsa and avocado.

Dinner:

- Grill vegetable kabobs, accompanied by wild rice.
- Steamed asparagus.

For dessert, baked pear with cinnamon.

Ensure also that in accordance with your liking, tastes, nutritional status and serving size, you modify in this menu plan. You can also introduce healthy snacks such as fresh fruits, raw vegetables or a few nuts in your daily eating plan. It is always advisable that you seek assistance of your doctor, nutritionist, or any health practitioner in this regard for personalized advice.

Monitoring progress and acknowledging health gains are important parts of any diet, like the Pritikin diet.

 Here's a guide to help beginners monitor their progress and understand the potential health benefits:

1. **Keep a Food Diary:**

- Keep a record of your daily food, drink, and snacks. Pay close attention to serving size, method of preparation in food and how you feel following your meal.

2. **Monitor Physical Changes:**
- Monitor your weight, body measurements, and fit of clothes. Always bear in mind that progress is not synonymous with weight loss alone.

3. **Energy Levels**:

- Ensure that you regulate your body's energy levels during the day. High energy levels may indicate that one has a balanced diet.

4. **Mood and Mental Clarity:**

- Document any variations in mood, attention or clarity of thought. Cognitive functioning can be enhanced by a balanced diet.

5. **Physical Activity:**

- Record your exercise routine. A healthy diet when combined with regular physical activity leads to good health. management journal.

6. **Sleep Quality:**

- Track your sleep patterns. Sleep quality can be improved by eating a healthy diet.

7. **Digestive Health:**

- Follow alterations in digestion and bowel motions. Eating a diets with fiber-rich foods such as fruits, vegetables, and whole grains promotes good digestion system.

8. Weight Management:

- For instance, the Pritikin diet, which is mainly high in whole foods, might help maintain appropriate nutrition as well as satisfactory intake that will aid in successful weight loss regimen.

9. Improved Heart Health:

- Low fat and cholesterol containing foods form the core of healthy diet, which when followed, may lead to lowered risk of diseases related to heart problem.

10. Better Blood Sugar Control:

- The Pritikin Diet includes whole grain foods and high fiber products, which may assist in controlling blood sugar for individuals with diabetes or prediabetes.

11. Better Blood Sugar Control:

- The Pritikin diet includes whole grains and fiber-rich products which are beneficial for people with diabetes as well as for those who are predisposed to it.

12.   **Reduced Inflammation:**

- Such a diet focuses on anti-inflammatory foods such as fruits, vegetables and omega-3 fatty acids that can reduce inflammation in the body.

13.   **Enhanced Nutrient Intake:**

- Eating different nutritional foods is healthy as it supplies useful vitamins, mineral and antioxidants.

14.   **Improved Lipid Profile:**

- Research studies have found that Pritikin Diet can improve lipid profiles such as lowering of LDL cholesterol and triglycerides.

15.   **Increased Satiety:**

- For instance, taking fiber with proteins contributes towards a sense of satiety, thus eliminating food cravings.

16.   **Balanced Blood Pressure:**

- In addition, a diet focusing on low sodium and high potassium helps in better blood pressure regulation.

Tips for Success:

1. **Be Consistent:**
- It is advisable to allow your body time to adjust to the new dietary habits. Long term success requires consistency.
2. **Celebrate Small Wins:**
- Celebrate what you have achieved and reward yourself even if you opt for a healthy snack or add vegetables to your diet.
3. **Stay Hydrated:**
- Take lots of water for general wellbeing and good digestion.
4. **Seek Support:**
- Get in touch with other people on diet, or health care giver or dietitian.

- It is advisable to have periodic consultation with a doctor to evaluate total health, which includes blood pressure reading, cholesterol levels, and other factors of significance.
- Note that there are many ways of reacting to certain diets. It is crucial that those with underlying health issues consult their physician before adopting such an approach.
- However not all of you will react in a similar way to the dietary changes. However, if you already have certain health problems or fear some of them, contact your doctor, they will give you individual recommendations and advices.

5. **Focus on Whole Foods**: Emphasize whole, unprocessed foods. Ensure that you use fruits, vegetables, whole grains, lean proteins, and legumes in preparing your meals.

6. **Stay Hydrated:** Drinking a lot of water throughout the day is also beneficial. Water is important for general well-being and may promote food intake and saturation.

7. **Choose Lean Proteins:** Choose lean protein supplies comprising fish, fowl, beans, and pulses. Limit red and processed meats.

8. Choose Lean Proteins: Choose lean protein supplies comprising fish, fowl, beans, and pulses. Limit red and processed meats.

Conclusion

Summing up, Pritikin diet is an attempt to promote cardio vasculature health and general life quality; it promotes reduced fat and increased fiber intake based on whole non-refined ingredients.

Here's a summary of key points for beginners:

1. **Focus on Whole Foods:** Eat meals based on whole foods like fruits, vegetables, whole grains, lean proteins, and legumes. These are high in nutrient and fiber-rich foods.

2. **Choose Lean Protein:** Go for lean proteins, chicken, fish, beans, and other legumes. Eat less red or processed meat.

3. **Limit Saturated and Trans Fats**: Minimize the usage or consumption of food products with high levels of saturated and trans fats like fried or commercial

4. **Limit Added Sugars**: Cut down on sugary foods and drinks. For a sweeter option, opt for fruit and other

5. **Exercise Regularly**: Have a nutritious diet coupled with daily exercise. Ensure incorporation of some aerobic activities along with the strength exercises in a way they complement each other for general well-being.

6. **Plan and Prepare Meals**: Ensure you plan your meals and cook them at home. You are in a much better position to control quality of ingredients and cooking processes.

7. **Educate Yourself:** Get familiar with Pritikin Diet's principles and find out what vitamins are contained in the various kinds of food. Such knowledge enables you make educated decisions.

8. **Consult with a Professional**: It is advisable that one should seek permission from a qualified healthcare professional or a registered dietitian before effecting any serious food changes, especially in case of some underlying ailments and health complications.

9. **Regular exercise**. combined with a nutritious diet, is essential for overall well-being. It's crucial to incorporate aerobic and strength exercises in a complementary manner.

Familiarize yourself with Pritikin Diet principles and understand the vitamins found in different food types to make informed decisions.

baked goods. Select healthier ways of cooking such as grilling and steaming.

Prioritize Fiber: Try to include high fiber foods in your diet such as wholegrain, fruits, vegetables, and legumes. Fiber is known to enhance fullness or satisfaction levels during eating, and it is very important for the normal functioning of the bowels.

Monitor Portion Sizes: Watch out on how much you eat as too much is not good. Use small plates on your table to assist with portion control.

Stay Hydrated: Ensure you take enough water every time. The body greatly needs water in order to stay healthy and it may also result to a sense of fullness which can suppress unnecessary snacks.